A Parent's Guide to Vision in Aut

Ian Jordan

ISBN 978-1-326-10938-7

Chapters

Acknowledgements   4

Introduction   5

Autism   9

Vision in autism   10

Accommodation and convergence   13

Health tests   17

Visual processing problems in autistic children   19

Development - Birth to school   26

Visual processing in ASD   28

Cognitive changes in ASD   40

Sensory integration   64

Synesthesia   69

Visual problems or visual processing problems?   70

Assessment techniques   75

The future   79

The author   80

Acknowledgements

This book was made possible by my wife, Beatrice, who not only has an extraordinary knowledge of vision in autism, but can achieve results with complex and difficult visual presentations which often astound me. She edited and made changes to the texts that have made extremely complex concepts readable for a parent. Many others have contributed, often more than they realise, thank you. I would like to thank the staff at Jordans in Ayr, Jenny Lynch, Janice Watson, Gillian Maclean, Margaret McCaw, In addition Sue Stephenson, Sally Ann Olivier, Win Wood, Paul Shattock, Paul Whitely, John Anderson, Graham Street, Carol Rutherford, Shona Linton, Mike Gilsennan, Robert Longhurst, Mike Charles, Sarah Brown and probably a thousand others.

The best teachers of all are the children themselves – I've learnt a lot from you – thank you

Introduction

It is assumed by many professionals and families that people that are on the autistic spectrum have similar vision to those who are not on the spectrum. This could not be further from the truth. This booklet is aimed principally at the parents of children on the spectrum, those on the spectrum themselves and professionals who want some basic knowledge of the problems which are faced.

Most people believe that other people perceive the world in a similar way to the way they themselves see it. Some may require spectacles to correct refractive errors but, in essence, what they see and how their bodies react to the visual input are very much the same for all individuals. But what if this assumption is incorrect? What if just about everything the child on spectrum sees can be fundamentally different from that of the general population? It would make the standard eye examination and standard interventions unsafe (although they may be suitable in some cases) and the training of the optical professional inadequate. It is obvious to me (and I suspect most parents and those with knowledge of the sensory processing problems that are so obvious in ASD) that the current optical model requires a fundamental rethink with regard to children (and adults) on the spectrum.

Research into vision and visual processing in ASD is poor. This is due to the way in which ASD is approached in respect to the current optical paradigm, and this, I believe is inappropriate. The diagnosis of autism is based on behaviours observed by a range of professionals and reported difficulties with communications. It does not look for the causes of these difficulties and when there are potentially numerous conditions which can cause symptoms it makes the diagnosis itself somewhat strange. It certainly means that research becomes immediately unreliable as it is quite possible that the research has been conducted on a number of conditions rather than the intended one. It also means interventions based on research may be completely inappropriate. It means that professionals must be trained to an adequate level in recognition of problems, how to assess and intervene and what the results of the interventions may be. Currently professional training is at best patchy and in some professions such as the optical professions – almost non-existent. Yet professionals often will often advise parents, even if they have virtually no knowledge, and even tell the parent that they are wrong in their ideas about their child. The parent is in general the expert on their own child and their views are valid (and often much better than those of the professional). There should always be a consensus and if it feels right to the parent, it usually is right. This applies particularly to vision and visual processing problems in autism. The effects are immediate and can be seen. If interventions work, the parent will usually see them, and so will the child, and so will the professional.

Professionals often jealously guard their position, even when their knowledge levels are limited. In autism this position makes them often make pronouncements that are difficult for the parent to believe and when queried, the professional may state that *they* are the expert and that the parent has to follow their recommendations.

To make matters worse we are seeing a disturbing trend. If a person disagrees with a professional they take the risk of being accused of fabrication of injury or illness (sometimes called Munchausen by proxy). Parental skills will often be called into question and it is not unknown for children to be removed from their families by a well-meaning system. This area is obviously controversial and in some rare cases a parent may be unsuitable, but in one week in our practice we had five parents that had been accused. It would beggar belief that it was true.

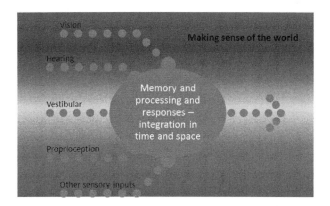

Autism

Autism is usually defined as a series of abnormal behaviours related to social communication The condition itself is not specified and may be one or a combination of problems ranging from fragile X or other genetic variations to a sensory processing disorder or even potentially brain damage. Immune problems, gut difficulties, biomedical and other physical problems have been implicated, making addressing the condition impossible from only a diagnosis. Further tests are required making the initial diagnosis a waste of time in many cases.

Until autism is divided into the numerous conditions it actually is and differentiated then research and intervention will always be problematical.

 A current diagnosis is almost completely useless in determining how to approach interventions.

It is by good fortune that some improve with interventions but it is of no surprise that the majority have a struggle.

Vision in autism

The standard eye test

Refractive problems (long sight, short sight, astigmatism) are found in ASD as in the rest of the community and it is important that they are assessed by an optometrist or ophthalmologist. However there are some significant differences between those on the spectrum and the general population which can be very important.

A significant proportion of children on the spectrum are hypersensitive and very small prescriptions found may be critical. Depth of focus can be extremely shallow and may at times be virtually non-existent. To make it more complicated the refractive error (prescription) can be very sensitive to visual stimulus in many cases and change power significantly depending on the environment. This problem is not only found in ASD - for example major prescription changes are often found due to light levels when night driving is a problem. A significant proportion of the population are bothered by this phenomenon and it may be responsible for some car accidents at night. A good optometrist will address this problem routinely in an eye test and undertake low light level testing when night driving is a problem.

On the other hand a very small number are incredibly insensitive to virtually every visual intervention and massive differences in prescription seem to make little difference.

Visual acuity is often a poor method of assessing performance for those on the spectrum as the visual problems experienced are often not elicited by reading a sight test chart (although some clues such as reading the letters out in the wrong order may give "pointers"). Often the child can see the bottom line of the chart when they have massive visual problems.

Standard use of drugs (eye drops) in the eye test can be very unpleasant for some of those on the spectrum as they may work unpredictably and what would be in normal circumstance be slightly uncomfortable may produce pain which may be extreme and persistent. Where possible they should be avoided but the professional has to judge when they are critical for the child and benefits outweigh the potential problems.

Normal eye testing criteria such as visual field testing using visual field instruments can give anomalous results as the visual field of the child may be dependent on the target being observed and the point target which is found in optometric instrumentation can produce very different results from other targets. In addition standard visual field tests may be difficult for an autistic child as the time taken in standard optometric field testing can be beyond the concentration span of the child. It is true that many children on the spectrum have visual field difficulties although it would not be standard procedure to assess these. Neglect (where the visual field is not interpreted correctly and it may be very blurred) is common and functional loss of the lower visual field is found in a high proportion of ASD children.

Accommodation and convergence

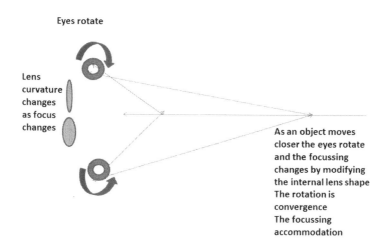

Eyes rotate

Lens curvature changes as focus changes

As an object moves closer the eyes rotate and the focussing changes by modifying the internal lens shape
The rotation is convergence
The focussing accommodation

The ability to focus on near objects (accommodation) is normally age dependent. You can just about predict the age of a person by their focussing ability (we all need reading spectacles in our late forties / early fifties). This is not true in ASD. It is usual for a subgroup to have much reduced accommodation causing some reading difficulties and problems with hand eye coordination. Standard optometric treatment is to give a prescription to reduce the need for accommodation but this may be inappropriate in ASD as the problem can be usually be addressed in better ways such as modifying stimulus.

Convergence is the ability of the eyes to rotate to fixate on a near object. Unequal convergence between the two eyes is common in autism and as fixation difficulties cause problems with tracking and hand eye coordination there are inevitably problems at school and in sport. Standard treatment may include exercises and prisms. However it is difficult to persuade a non-verbal autistic child to do exercises and others won't because of the discomfort and difficulties with comprehension. Prisms may be appropriate but may be difficult to prescribe as feedback may be limited. Stimulus control may be more appropriate.

Strabismus (squint) and amblyopia (lazy eye)

A high proportion of those on the spectrum may present with a strabismus (where two eyes do not fuse images correctly and one eye moves to a misaligned position to enable the brain to deal with the images). In angle of this misalignment varies from virtually imperceptible to an obvious "turn" in the eye. It may be a constant turn or it may be variable or alternating.

What causes a strabismus? Is it muscle problems, image size differences, refractive errors or control mechanisms? Some squints caused by refractive error respond well to standard treatment (which are probably best addressed optically with contact lenses – spectacles may introduce image size problems but are easier and less expensive - but I sympathise with anyone trying to fit a child who does not want a contact lens in his eye!). Others are treated surgically (often for cosmetic reasons) but few are treated for timing or image size difficulties although when they are remarkable and immediate results are possible.

Amblyopia (when one eye sees significantly less well than the other) is usually treated in the UK by occluding (covering up with a patch) the good eye in the hope that by using the blurred eye it will start working. Although this method is considered best practice in the UK there is a significant number of professionals (particularly abroad) who would consider it inappropriate and that other methods are better. My own position is that when acuity can be improved immediately in the "bad eye" using other techniques then it may be that occlusion is inappropriate. However techniques that can achieve this are rarely used in the UK.

Health tests

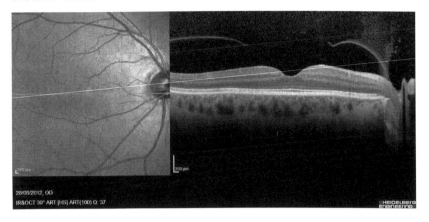

Using an OCT may be the best method of checking the health of the eyes of a visually hypersensitive child.

It is absolutely essential that children's eyes are tested as early as possible whether they are on the spectrum or not. In general, the earlier eye problems are addressed, the better. The youngest person tested in our practice was only six days old, but this was because of a family history of autism with complex visual difficulties.

There are a variety of tests that can be done to check the eye health of children on the spectrum. To the best of my knowledge there is no greater risk of eye disease for children on the spectrum.

It is possible to test a non-verbal or non-cooperative child although it is more difficult and results may be slightly less accurate.

Visual processing problems in autistic children

Processing of visual information in ASD is however very different. Standard visual tests are inadequate to determine what the child is experiencing and a completely different approach is necessary.

Whilst I am explaining how we approach problems in our practice, it is perfectly acceptable to approach these problems in a different way. The methods are not fixed and my own opinion is that as every child on the spectrum presents differently they should be flexible. To improve on what we do is desirable (we are well aware that this is a developing field and as new knowledge expands the paradigm – it is inevitable that the methods used should change). I hope that the challenge will be taken up and the techniques we use are rendered obsolete by improvement.

Signs and symptoms

We prefer to separate the child from the parent at some point. This enables us to get a parental view without little ears trying to second guess how to answer. The child is also initially assessed using standard optometric procedures including questioning to establish their ideas of their visual problems, an initial refraction, binocular vision tests, stereopsis (many on the spectrum have poor 3D vision), confrontational visual fields, visual acuities, accommodation and convergence. We may use optical coherence tomography to look at the retina (the back of the eye) as it is often preferable to standard ophthalmoscopy for the child who is hyper-sensitive to light. Eye drops are often cruel to the child on the spectrum and we avoid using them whenever possible.

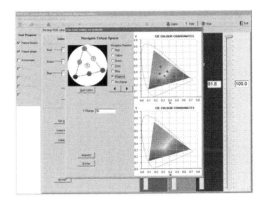

Assessing stimulus is very scientific

The way the child reacts during the test may also be important e.g. how they read the chart. Is confusion present? The verbal child will often be extremely precise in their comments and will answer the questions well. Non-verbal children can be tested too although understanding their opinions may a problem. Makaton or various signing can be useful and it is remarkable how often we can communicate if a little imagination is used. Use of puppets and third person evaluation is sometimes helpful. Sometimes children speak for the first time in the practice and this always causes tears from the parents (we usually join in too!)

The child will also be observed. We would normally look at the gait, head position, listen to the speech, look at hand eye coordination and be aware of their behaviour – are they stimming for instance – and if so what are the stims doing in relation to their vision. Tics will be observed and addressed where possible.

The parent will be asked for a full history, symptoms and their opinions. These are crucial in ASD and the professional who disregards the parents' point of view loses much. In fact I suspect that in ASD it is impossible to take the family out of the assessment without seriously compromising it. We will look into the family background as some genetic influences are important in the assessment.

What we are interested in family background

History of migraine / epilepsy.

If there is a history of epilepsy or migraine it is common to find that similar problems manifest themselves in the child. Around a quarter of those on the spectrum may be epileptic and others may show frontal headaches or migraines. In addition comorbid difficulties with jaw control (grinding of teeth or involuntary biting of cheeks or tongues), dry mouths and eyes (children are often seen rubbing them particularly when reading), problems with high pitched sound, hair sensitivities (manifested as intolerance to haircuts) and some types of stomach pain may be found.

Allergies and sensitivities.

Allergies and sensitivities are common and may be associated with abnormal responses to medication. It is prudent to consider whether immune system difficulties are present. Many children on the spectrum are atopic (suffer hay fever, asthma, eczema) and food sensitivities are often present. Increased mucus production (snotty nose / glue ear) may indicate sensitivity. The most common is to milk or gluten and it is not unusual to see significant visual performance improvements if the diet is changed.

Gut problems – particularly irritable bowel or leaky gut.

There is now a substantial body of evidence linking autism with gut problems. However, this is controversial and it is beyond the scope of this book to go further. But if your child is suffering from gut problems and is autistic it may be a good idea to look into it yourself.

Previous visual problems.

Some visual problems may be inherited and therefore may have been passed down to the autistic child. It can be particularly difficult if there is both a visual problem and a visual processing problem associated with autism as symptoms may become more complex.

We then need to know a little about the pregnancy and birth as problems before and around the time of birth have been associated with autism and some of the symptoms that may be seen. It has been suggested that high stress levels in the mother or fever may be a factor. At birth there have been suggestions that C-sections may increase the risk of ASD. Some visual processing symptoms found in ASD may be caused by oxygen deprivation around birth although this has not been conclusively proved.

There is a difference in the ratio of autism development in recent times. In the past the majority of autism presentations were found from birth and relatively few were cases of regression. This ratio sems to have changed although the causes are not clear but they are likely to be due to some common factors in the environment. There have been numerous papers and each seems to suggest a different cause, but this may reflect the fact that there are a large number of causes or that the causes are inter-related.

The prevalence of ASD seems to be increasing at an alarming rate. Even allowing for better detection, numbers have increased massively. Society is complacent – but when the inevitable bills start to roll in, things will have to change. We need to address problems as early as possible and therefore we have to recognise risk factors in development.

Autism prevalence increase

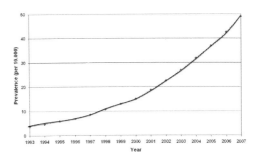

Development - Birth to school

Development from birth is important as there are a number of difficulties directly associated with ASD.

These include "loose ligaments", gut problems (including constipation / diarrhoea, bloating, reflux), a "floppy" baby, late talking and walking (with, controversially, possible problems with retained reflexes). Immune problems are considered by many to be related to ASD and a significant minority of people are concerned that vaccination or other medications may be a factor.

Regression is common, usually at around a year to eighteen months of age. The reason why regression occurs is not known and there are a number of potential causes. The arguments are complex and beyond this booklet.

Diagnosis is possible at this time but it is rarely given in the UK unless the problems are profound. In some countries diagnosis takes place very early (such as Israel in which very early diagnosis is common). From now on diagnosis may take place but where you live may influence this. It is best to get a diagnosis as early as possible as educational establishments may require it before taking action.

At the age of around three years the child will start nursery. In most cases they will have some difficulties with social interaction and in a good nursery this will be recognised and interventions will be put in place.

Obviously decisions will need to be made as to the best education for the child. There are many factors to take into account before the decision is taken, one of which is how the child responds to sensory input. The child usually does not recognize that their sensory input is unusual – but the visual world of autism often surprises the parent and sometimes even shocks.

Visual processing in ASD

Visual processing problems are very common and perhaps as many as nine out of ten children on the spectrum have some problems. These vary from minor difficulties to horrendous problems which make life extraordinarily difficult. There is a wide range of difficulties which may be encountered, ranging from straightforward difficulties with visual symptoms, to complex problems which may not appear to have any obvious visual complications but are in fact major and convoluted visual anomalies.

Tinted lenses are usually the best and sometimes the only method of treating visual processing problems. Although tints and filters may appear to be a simple intervention they are in fact extremely complex and it needs a great deal of knowledge to be able to determine the range of filters that are suitable for a variety of lighting conditions. Not all tints and filters are the same – even if they look identical. Training is very limited even in the professions that most members of the public would expect to be experts with some very significant consequences for those on the autistic spectrum. It is for instance virtually impossible to prescribe accurately using trial and error and lens matching colours by eye is only possible to a limited degree. It may surprise people that standards and tolerances are not specified even though they could be (standards in colour have been around since the 1930's but the optical professional training has ignored this inconvenient truth for accurate tint prescribing)

It is a fact that the only people in the UK who can prescribe clinical tints or dispense spectacles with a prescription to children are optometrists (prescribe and dispense) and opticians (dispense – although they are usually the person to decide on the filter). They therefore have a duty of care to recognise when they are necessary, determine the optimum filter and dispense it accurately. They should know the effects of the tint and filter and how to modify it if necessary. Currently the training in this area is minimal and is not considered to be important by many in the professions.

Types of visual processing problem

Visual processing problems fall into a number of types

Timing problems

Mapping and control difficulties

Cognitive complications

Sensory integration problems

Synesthetic anomalies

Most eye examinations (with some notable exceptions) will not address visual processing problems even though the only person who can prescribe tints for clinical need legally is the optometrist! Obviously there may be legal implications, but these have yet to be tested.

Timing

It has been known since 1922 that visual processing speed can be modified by changing visual stimulus. The principle is completely accepted although it is rarely addressed by the medical or optical professions.

Timing problems are very common in ASD. I estimate that at least three quarters of those on the spectrum have some difficulties. For the most part these are ignored.

Visual processing speed difficulties can be addressed by using properly prescribed filters. Timing can be tuned extremely accurately if the optical professional has adequate instrumentation and sufficient knowledge.

Types of timing problem

The most obvious problem is the Pulfrich phenomenon. When the vision from one eye is processed at a different speed from that of the other, there are a number of effects. The first is that space appears to twist and as a consequence there are problems with sport, movement and distortion of image. Sometimes double vision and / or strabismus may result. Speed of movement may be difficult to determine particularly with objects crossing the visual field. In addition there will be inevitable clumsiness and as a consequence safety issues need to be considered.

Although the Pulfrich effect is common it is rarely recognised during the eye test partly due to the static rather than dynamic nature of the refractive process. The best intervention is using tinted spectacles or in some cases contact lenses. However, the appearance of the spectacles may be a problem as it is often necessary to have a different colour or density in each eye. Complex prescribing techniques can sometimes get around this problem but that is beyond the scope of this booklet.

Timing problems between central and peripheral vision may be present in ASD. This may produce difficulties in understanding what is going on in the classroom and clumsiness when walking around (the area of clear visual field may be very small). Bleaching of the peripheral field is sometimes found. Road safety will be compromised and it is likely that the child will have a tendency to walk into things such as door frames or furniture.

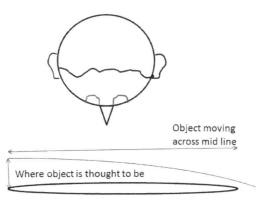

The Pulfrich effect – top track shows real object, real movement
bottom two tracks – where object may appear to be seen

Object moving across mid line

Where object is thought to be

However it is likely the child may be able to see the bottom line of the sight test chart and the optometrist may not be aware of the major visual problem that is present.

Integration of vision with other sensory systems assumes that they are synchronous i.e. processed at the same time. When the timing of visual processing is not in synch with the other sensory systems then it is essential that vision is tuned in time to prevent problems. The effects of desynchronised senses in ASD can be profound. I believe that any optical professional should be able to synchronise visual timing – providing they have adequate instrumentation. The most obvious problem of desynchronicity is with the miss-timing of hearing with vision.

When hearing people speak is desynchronised with vision there are a number of potential effects in ASD. The most obvious is for a child to have difficulties looking at someone's face when they are speaking. When lip synch is out it is difficult to maintain focus (it's a bit like watching a film that is out of synch – you can do it – but it's not pleasant) and is easier to look away. The teacher who says "look at me while I am talking to you!" may be making it impossible for a child to listen as they cannot do both at the same time. A lesser known effect of desynchronisation is that of the McGurk effect. This can change the sound of word perception and in some cases cause major problems with comprehension. A possible consequence of this is that that mimicry can be difficult and therefore speech can be affected. When vision and hearing are in time the child is aware of how they are speaking and can start to speak normally. In rare cases where there is overload of information being processed, the lips and/or the voice may seem to freeze making it impossible to process information.

Sounds may be desynchronised making positional knowledge a problem that can result in risks in the street as transport sounds may not warn of a vehicle's approach.

Checking timing of vision with hearing is very easy and the effects are obvious both to the child and parent.

A further form of desynchronised vision with senses is that with touch. When this happens it can have devastating consequences. A child may not know where their body is relative to the environment. It causes falls (injuries are common), praxis (planning and execution of movement) difficulties which impacts on writing and movement. Visual feedback has to coincide with body positional awareness. It often doesn't in ASD. Again it is easy to check and resolve by modifying visual input by changing its timing.

Mapping and control problems

We assume that other people see things in the same sequence as we do. This is not necessarily the case in ASD. If we think of the world as a map, everything can be specified in a position defined by its X/Y coordinates. In ASD these coordinates may be in the wrong position on the map! In other words the visual map may show things to be in the wrong position. In reading, this effect is common in ASD – the letters or words may displace, change sequence or in extreme cases may appear to fall off the page!. In addition the object may be inverted or rotated. This is common in reading where letters reverse and invert (d/b p/b). In some cases part of the map may disappear. This is reflected in parts of the words or letters disappearing from the text. In some cases the reference grid becomes distorted resulting in magnification changes and crowding of letters or words. Alternatively spaces may appear in the wrong places or become changed in dimensions. These symptoms cause major problems in reading and must be resolved using visual techniques - educational interventions are not appropriate. Dyslexia is a common consequence and it is not appropriate to use language based interventions when it is a visual problem causing the language difficulty.

In rare cases the map will spin and this produces the strange phenomenon of words and letters rotating. In other cases parts of the map may appear more than once giving the impression of double vision. There are a number of variations of this including an annulus (a bit like a doughnut effect) in which the double vision image is changed in size (causing complex diplopia which would not normally be picked up in an eye test). Others types of double vision include those in which part of the map may replicate causing image fragmentation. (Again this will not be observed in an eye test). Physiological diplopia during convergence (the double vision caused by eyes looking at a close object and becoming crossed) can be addressed extremely well using filters and will usually stop immediately. It is common in ASD. Any double vision must be assessed by an optical professional as other more serious causes, although very rare, must be discounted.

Distortion such as keystone (when objects appear to tilt away from or towards the viewer) may be present in the map – and this may resolve with prisms or in some cases stimulus control.

The body awareness map of a child on the spectrum is often poor in that they have never built up the visual map of position in association with the proprioceptive (positional) and vestibular (balance and head position) maps. They do not always know where their body is, or where and when it has been touched. In extreme cases perception can be wildly inaccurate and cause the child major problems.

Adequate mapping is the basis for much movement control. We have a projected image of ourselves in relation to space around us and it is usually this knowledge that enables us to direct the body. Without this knowledge our eyes may not move to the correct place and limbs may not move correctly. Changing visual stimulus will often produce marked and obvious effects to gait, hand eye coordination and visual tracking in reading. Sport can be affected massively by this effect even up to elite level (we have a number of world and national champions who benefit from visual processing control interventions).

In some cases the muscles around the eye cause the eye to rotate, and objects to tilt and twist. This too responds to visual stimulus control although the mechanism is not clear. It often manifests itself by a child rotating a book when reading or writing to maintain the appearance of vertical / horizontal text.

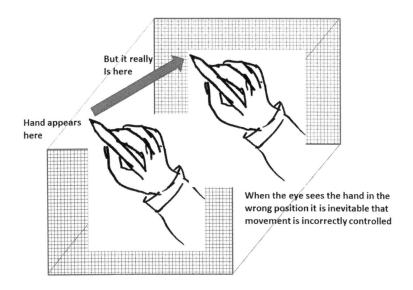

But it really is here

Hand appears here

When the eye sees the hand in the wrong position it is inevitable that movement is incorrectly controlled

Cognitive changes in ASD

There are many cognitive differences in autism. The greatest problem experienced by many on the spectrum is that of recognition of faces and expressions. Can you imagine a life in which you cannot recognize your mother, wife, husband, children and friends? Worse than that, the faces you look at may cause you physical pain, may appear to be monsters or look aggressively at you. You have never even seen yourself in a mirror – or what you do see is disturbing. Faces may detach from their body, change to a different animal or distort. The world can be terrifying. You think you are going mad! And in many cases the response of your parent or teacher is –" look me in the eye when I am talking to you!" It must appear that they are very cruel.

We now know of a large number of facial recognition and expression recognition problems.

The good news

NEARLY ALL TYPES OF FACIAL RECOGNITION DIFFICULTIES RESPOND WELL TO TREATMENT WITH PROPERLY PRESCRIBED FILTERS

The bad news

The optical professions are not trained to address this problem. I believe this to be unacceptable as the results are extraordinarily good and easy to achieve.

Types of facial recognition problem

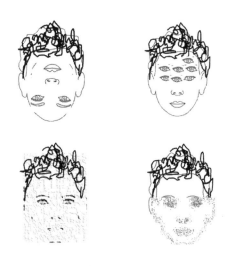

Common facial appearance changes seen in autism

Flattening of facial features

There is an appearance of age reduction – wrinkles appear to flatten

Occasionally the person viewed may appear to change gender – usually male to female.

Dysmorphia (perception of the persons own body parts may be incorrect)

In extreme cases faces become cartoon-like and have little or no contours consistent with a form of 3D visual fusion problem. As the depth of features within the face appears to change– comments include "the nose appears to stick out", "the face becomes 3D". This type of 3D effect does not appear when looking at other objects and is not found using optometric 3D testing methods.

All cases have resolved immediately with stimulus control intervention

Deepening of features - the opposite effect of that above

Age appears to increase and wrinkles become deeper and more apparent. With intervention the person becomes younger looking. In rare cases cartoons seen on television or in the cinema may appear as real people.

All cases to date have resolved with optimum stimulus.

Loss of visual field

The most common loss is a contralateral hemianopia (loss of half the field when looking at a face in each eye) which inevitably results in convergence difficulties. This may be causative of strabismus as fusion is impossible. Stimulus treatment will resolve symptoms immediately. Professional assessment is essential as there can be other causes which can be of major importance.

Attentional field loss is common in ASD (perhaps the most common difficulty). This results in a small area of clear vision, with an annular blurred area which becomes progressively more blurred peripherally. This effect would not show up in a standard visual field assessment as standard optometric instrumentation would still reveal light sensitivity. It causes facial and expression recognition problems and if it is present when walking (this is not a symptom just found in face viewing) then it can make moving around hazardous. It will always impact on spatial awareness and clumsiness in general.

When looking at a face, insufficient information is processed without using scanning – moving the eyes around the face to work out features and expression. Scanning is however too slow to enable adequate expression processing and it is inevitable that difficulties are found. Behavioural interventions are inevitably poor. Field restoration is immediate with stimulus modification. The face instead of being clear in a small area is changed to the whole face being visible without scanning. Hemianopias (loss of half the visual field) and quadrant field loss can resolve immediately resulting in improvement in eye movement and fixation.

Attentional field loss has been resolved in all cases to date and peripheral blurring appears to become clear. Faces described as only having a small area clear become fully clear. This is crucial in ASD as it will allow the whole face to be seen at the same time and consequent facial recognition and expression / mood recognition becomes possible.

Loss of features in the face

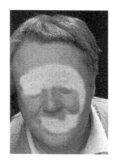

Features within the face may disappear from view. Insufficient facial information may be present for processing. Whilst superficially similar to a field loss it may be that the processing of a particular area of face regardless of position is lost and therefore it is not angle dependent. Restoration of facial features is crucial to facial and expression recognition. In some cases a dorsal stream or ventral stream difficulty may also exist. Symptoms have resolved in virtually all cases by providing the optimum stimulus.

Distortion

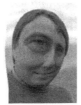

The face may appear to twist, distort or change shape. It may appear to melt. It is often described as being similar to the images seen in a "hall of mirrors" or it may be describes as the face "melts" or the mouth becomes like a clown. It can be very disturbing. Symptoms have resolved (in all cases to date) with stimulus modification and distortion is no longer reported.

Movement related blurring

Faces may only be blurred during movement. This may involve persistence (where the face moves yet the image of where it has been remains)motion, blurring or blending of information. In some cases the speed of movement and direction may be critical. This may also apply to the person moving so they only have difficulties with movement relative to themselves. Flicker and edge recognition problems e.g. steps / stair ascending / descending, or patterns in wallpapers or text are often found. There may be a relationship with trigeminal nerve difficulties.

It has resolved with lenses in all cases to date.

Lip synch

Timing of visual information is often at a different time from hearing the spoken word. The McGurk effect, in which speech is perceived as distorted is common. The effect of desynchronised vision with speech may be diagnosed as an auditory processing difficulty or a communication problem but if there is a visual component it will often resolve immediately. This is very common in ASD and must be addressed in order to stop unpleasant symptoms.

A vectored Pulfrich intervention (a type of visual stimulus control) may be used to synchronise vision and sound. This can have profound effects. Results have been immediate in all cases to date and symptoms are no longer perceived or they are drastically reduced.

Arousal level in the brain changes with filters

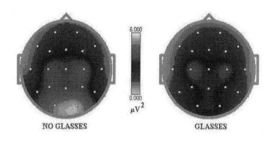

With acknowledgements to Dr B Steffert and Prof Y Kropitov

Synesthetic effects

Synaesthesia is where one sense is interpreted as another.

Crossed sensory interpretation with facial viewing is rare – when seen it usually presents as a sound or as pain, although tastes and smells have also been reported. A reverse effect can often be seen in which facial features may be modified by pressure on the hands or on focal points on the forehead. Tuning of visual stimulus with the synesthetic effect has up to now resolved all symptoms. It is unlikely that this will always be the case as there are many forms of synaesthesia which do not appear to be related to vision. This area needs significant research as it is of crucial importance in ASD and yet it is an almost unknown entity, even to experts.

Features appearing to float in air

A rare effect is in which features in the face detach and appear to be seen in mid-air adjacent to the face. The face itself appears to be flat and featureless. This strange effect can be resolved using stimulus control although the mechanism is unknown. We have only seen two cases, both of which resolved immediately with stimulus change.

Faces causing pain

In a form of synaesthesia, looking at a face may provoke discomfort or pain. It is often essential to look away. Pain is usually perceived in the forehead or in the eye area. Itchiness in the area of the eye, and dry eye or mouth (child may drink a lot of water) may be experienced. Refractive problems may play a part in this as presbyopia, hypermetropia, and astigmatism are common in those reporting this symptom, yet myopic patients very rarely experience it.

Pain may move to a different focal point such as the ear lobe, change its feeling to a different form such a sharp pain changing to throbbing and eventually disappear with stimulus modification. Other pain that may be found in ASD may also stop when this is addressed although the mechanism is unclear.

Faces turning to animals / other objects

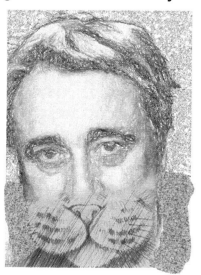

Faces changing appearance to that of an animal is a relatively common symptom and we estimate that at least 5% of those on the autistic spectrum will describe this symptom – although they usually will not volunteer it as they often think that they are going mad!

A range of animals has been reported from giraffes to spiders. In one case only, one side of the face appeared to change (to a hamster) and the other remained human. The most common animals seen are cats although a large number of other animals have been described. A small number of birds have been described (interestingly they have all been raptors – and the person being viewed has a "big nose" described – so there may be some associative effects)

A rare variation is that of a face changing to a plant such as broccoli (we have only seen two cases of this). A more common metamorphosis is to see faces change to monsters. This can be terrifying and is often the cause of refusal to enter a classroom. Imagine when you got to class and your classmates appeared as ghouls. I think anyone would be scared.

It is not surprising that children have a natural reluctance to report symptoms for fear of ridicule – their parents will often say ," don't be silly" if they report it. It is easier to remain silent. It can be a very disturbing or terrifying experience.

Resolution of effect appears to be universal with stimulus control. We can also provoke this symptom by reversing the stimulus control.

Faces changing colour

Monochromatic faces may be perceived (faces becoming one colour). This has been associated with drug or alcohol intake but this is not always so. Faces have been described as "Smurf-like" or resembling the "Incredible Hulk" This is a self- resolving symptom in all cases to date although speed of resolution may be measured in hours.

In other rare cases faces become striped, pixelated or appear to be in monochrome blocks as though they are an impressionist painting. These symptoms have resolved using stimulus control to date but we have only seen small numbers.

Faces changing size

Faces may become enormous or tiny. Sometimes parts of the face such as the forehead or eyes may appear much larger whilst the rest of the face may remain the same size (fish eye effect). This effect is often very disturbing and upsetting. Stimulus control modification appears to be very successful in resolving this effect in all cases to date.

Diplopia / polyplopias

Double vision or multiple images are common. There are a number of manifestations seen. The most common is multiple component parts of the face e.g. multiple eyes, noses, mouths. They may be displaced horizontally, vertically or both. Sometimes they may be a result of persistence on head rotation. Sometimes peripheral vision is double during fixation (physiological diplopia). Multiple images can resolve immediately with stimulus control although there is always the possibility of fixation or muscle balance problems. These are checked before filters are assessed in all cases to rule out a binocular vision problem.

Faces inverting

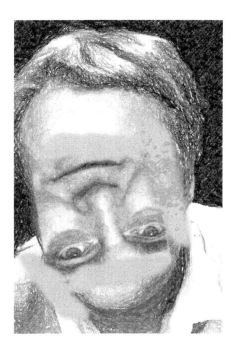

A rare symptom is that of faces appearing to turn upside down. The face appears to be the same shape but the features appear inverted – the hair may be still in the same position or inverted.

We have seen one child the patient would see the face rotated through 90 degrees, but 15 degrees is more common. I suspect that there are different mechanisms depending on rotation but as with many areas of facial recognition, we just don't know.

A rare inversion is when the patient describes the face as appearing to project inwards rather than out. The face has flipped to the correct orientation immediately with appropriate stimulus in all cases to date.

Bleaching

Features may completely bleach and disappear – this may be a permanent feature and is often described as face blindness. The hair and body and other objects do not disappear.

Appropriate stimulus control is almost invariably successful. The emotional effect of seeing faces for the first time is usually overwhelming and can cause distress at what has been missed. Sometimes it causes anger that a simple intervention could have been put in place by the optical community (had they been aware of it).

Persistence

Sometimes when the face moves it appears to be in two places at the same time. In extreme cases the persistence may be for a considerable time and it may actually be used in portrait painting by some artists. This may involve memory rather than pure persistence however. Immediate cessation of symptoms and improvement in the clarity of vision has been achieved with stimulus control. This also applies to the long period of persistence seen by some artists making it more likely that it is a persistence effect rather than use of memory.

Memory problems

Facial memories can be a problem i.e. the person cannot remember faces. Sometimes it can be that the face is remembered but the name is not. These problems are relatively common.

Stimulus control appears to have a very limited effect on purely memory related facial recognition difficulties. However it is often the case that what is perceived as a memory difficulty is in fact an inability to see the face properly in the first place. It is therefore prudent to rule this out.

Personal facial knowledge

Recognising your own face can be a problem in ASD. Your features are known from self-examination using touch but when looking in the mirror they may appear to be completely different.

Not being able to recognise one -self is a terrific handicap and has major effects on self-esteem. For girls in particular the belief that they may look like a monster is debilitating.   Optimum stimulus control can enable virtually everyone to see their own face. It can be very emotional when people see their own faces for the first time. Comments like "I thought I was a freak – until now" are common. Confidence, self- image and demeanour are regulated at least in part by own face recognition. This is one of the most important interventions (if not the most important) in ASD.

Mimicry

Mimicry relies on ability to see other faces and reproduce the facial expression on one's own. When the child is having facial expression problems they may appear angelic or expressionless. A further problem can be that the child is not aware of their own facial expression – their muscles controlling their face movements are not recognised. Improved mimicry relies on the ability to see other faces and be in control over their own. It follows that facial recognition is critical in developing personal facial expression.

Eye contact

Eye contact may cause pain, discomfort and be very difficult for those with problems. In virtually every case eye contact is normal or much improved with appropriate stimulus. However the person being viewed often finds it more difficult as they may not see the eyes of the viewer due to the tint obscuring the viewer's eyes due to spectral absorption. It is not unknown for the person with facial recognition difficulties to be asked to remove the tinted lenses because people without problems find it difficult to deal with a person looking at them with tinted spectacles.

Gestalt (the whole picture)

Sometimes the face becomes detached from the background – the background may disappear and the face may become effectively the whole attentional field. This is a very rare effect. It is not known whether stimulus control has an effect on this phenomenon.

Capgrass syndrome

Capgrass syndrome is a very rare anomaly in which the observer believes the person observed is an phoney "you look like my mother – but you are not – you are an imposter!". We have seen only one case of this which appeared to have been resolved with a refractive correction. It is not known whether this is affected by stimulus.

Freezing

Facial movement (usually mouth) may appear to freeze when observing someone speaking. The speech sound may appear to freeze or alternatively it may continue. This is a rare effect. Stimulus control appears to stop this effect, but as only small numbers have been seen with this problem, it is possible that results are idiosyncratic.

Heads detaching from body

This uncommon symptom has been characterised by the head following the body (being processed at a slower speed than the body). In all cases we have seen, the head appears to be distorted and eventually joins the body when movement stops. Movement processing anomalies such as the Pulfrich effect and mid line dominance problems are usually found. Stimulus control appears to stop this unpleasant and scary symptom, but numbers seen with this phenomenon are few.

Shadows

Shadows may be "seen" of bodies when none are present. This appears to be a form of hallucination or false memory. Stimulus control seems to have little effect on this symptom.

Hallucinations

Hallucinations are often reported (although again there is a tendency not to tell parents) ranging from seeing people from a TV programme appearing in the room at a later date to seeing people (mainly children) in either modern or old fashioned dress. Some children say they see ghosts! The mechanisms for these phenomena are not known and the discussion is beyond the scope of this booklet.

Visual echolalia

Faces previously seen may reappear within the current images being observed. Stimulus control appears to be extremely successful in stopping this rare symptom – but as it is uncommon this cannot be considered definitive.

Provoked effects

Provoking facial changes is possible for most that exhibit visual processing symptoms and for a significant proportion of people that do not, by the simple matter of providing inappropriate stimulation. Most, but not all symptoms (memory related symptoms do not seem to be provocable this way) are provocable in around 10% of the population. As lighting appears to provoke unpleasant symptoms, and filters reduce symptoms, it is clear that the environment may be critical in symptom provocation.

Amblyopia

Visual processing problems are much more common in eyes with reduced acuity (between 6/9 and 6/18). Congenital cataract has been cited as a marker for prosopagnosia (Duchaine) but this may be the acuity drop rather than the cataract. Reduced acuity appears to make facial processing more difficult.

Crowding phenomena in hyperopic eyes may also play a part. If stimulus control improves facial recognition then acuity will also be improved. However, reversing the stimulus modification will make symptom provocation / increase more likely

Related problems

Other objects may also appear to change shape, size or colour or become amorphous. The world can be a strange place for those on the spectrum. Nothing seen can be trusted.

This compounds with other sensory processing difficulties such as auditory processing disorders, sensory defensive]ness, modulation of sensory processing, vestibular and proprioceptive difficulties....

We normally rely on the veracity of information being inputted to our sensory systems, it being processed through matching and memory, and then action being taken as a response to this stable sensory world. In ASD this can be totally wrong, the sensory world is not as expected and does not match, and, the outputs do not respond in the way expected. Sensory processing problems are endemic in autism – and often cause the greatest difficulties.

Sensory integration

Bringing all the senses together can be an extremely complex task for those on the spectrum. For some it is impossible and they can only use one or sometimes two at the same time. Yet this is the way in which we understand the world – we rely on how we understand our sensory input. When we can't trust it or it overwhelms us, it is no wonder that meltdowns happen. A high proportion of the problems experienced by people on the spectrum are sensory, yet they are not prioritised. The earlier they are addressed, the better. Vision can affect all the sensory systems, and the effects can be profound.

Vision with hearing / vestibular

Vision can be used to eliminate or reduce auditory processing difficulties with immediate effect. It is prudent to consider cross over interventions at an early stage.

Parents should watch out for a child who responds to conversation or a question with a "what" or appears to switch off. Speech problems or unusual accents may also indicate a visual / auditory integration problem. In the UK an American accent in a British child may indicate a visual processing problem!

Auditory hyper/ hypo sensitivity – visual stimulus can be tuned to change perceived auditory volume. This may be a magnocellular effect.

Auditory processing speed – often children on the spectrum may perceive fast speaking as an incomprehensible jumble. This is related to visual persistence (where moving objects leave a trail) which is seen in many children in ASD. Treat the visual persistence and immediately the auditory persistence problems will cease in most cases.

Amblyopia (lazy eye) is often associated with an auditory processing problem generally described as poor hearing. Usually the same ear is affected as eye unless the child is cross lateral (where dominance is mixed between right and left depending on task), in which case it will be the opposite ear. Normal treatment is to patch the good eye (this sometimes affects the hearing too!). Using optimum filters (where appropriate) will usually improve the vision immediately and the hearing will improve at the same time.

Tinnitus is less common in ASD but responds extremely well to stimulus control. Results are very good in children – it usually resolves during the assessment of stimulus control.

Balance may be affected in unusual ways in ASD. Normally speaking posturography shows that closing eyes produces less stability but in some on the spectrum it can be better stability. This suggests that balance problem may be provoked by the visual input of the child.

Typically those on the spectrum have walking problems. They may tip toe, crab to one side or have difficulties with perception of the ground. In some cases these problems resolve immediately when using filters.

In another vestibular problem found in autism, dizziness may be felt during convergence – typically when reading. Filters will almost always resolve problems immediately.

Touch, pressure, temperature

Touch and pressure anomalies may also have a visual component in ASD. For those on the spectrum who find their pressure sensation is mixed up between deep and light pressure (child needs deep pressure in hugs, but finds discomfort in light touch e.g. seams of clothes, haircuts) stabilising visual processing will switch neural pathways and the symptoms will immediately cease. Weight perception (how heavy an individual feels) can also be affected.

Position and timing of touch are also aberrant for many on the spectrum with touch position felt in a different position and at a different time from that perceived visually. This can cause many problems to the child and it is essential that it is resolved. Stimulus control can tune this and therefore reduce the risk of problems due to not being aware of space

Pain awareness is often aberrant in ASD. This is a protective mechanism and when it is abnormal it can put the child in danger. It is crucial that it is addressed. It appears that visual processing modification can "normalise" pain perception in many cases.

Pressure problems are almost always associated with difficulties with temperature recognition (wearing wrong clothes, wanting a very hot / cold bath). Again this may be stabilised by visual stimulus control and changes are immediate.

Taste and smell

Taste and smell can be affected to a significant extent by visual stimulus control. The mechanism is unclear.

Dietary problems may have a visual processing component. A Dry mouth can be a sign of visual processing problems.

Texture of foods in the mouth and the swallow and gagging reflexes can be changed using vision. We can even have success in getting people to eat green vegetables! (But not all the time)

Synesthesia

Synesthesia is common in ASD yet is rarely recognised. It is where one sense is interpreted as another. This causes great problems for professionals. Do we address the cause or the effect – and do we know what the causative symptoms are, and what the effect is? It is extremely difficult to tell in some cases, particularly when there are multiple crossovers. In general terms we feel the best answer is to address as much as possible and maybe one of the interventions will be causative. But this is not a precise art. Maybe in the future we will be more accurate.

But it is extremely important to realise that provocation of symptoms can be the result of either not addressing the problem or by inappropriate stimulus. Whilst we address synaesthesia in practice I am acutely aware of the potential complications, but I suspect that anyone dealing with these complex problems will have significant difficulties.

Visual problems or visual processing problems?

There are many types of visual problem that are a direct result of processing difficulties. These give many symptoms some of which may be similar to refractive difficulties (but refractive correction will not resolve processing problems leading to problems such as non-tolerance of spectacles and poor performance). Those with visual processing problems may appear to have anomalous colour vision in tests such as the Ishihara but this may be due to crowding rather than true colour vision problems. Visual acuity (how well your child can see down a chart) may be misleading as responses do not necessarily determine how well a child can process visual information. They may see the bottom line of the chart yet have profound visual problems. Conversely a child who cannot see the chart well at all may only be experiencing minor difficulties. However they may not appreciate what they are missing.

Visual fields (how much you can see to the side and up and down when looking straight ahead) are commonly constricted (reduced) for those on the spectrum

Quite often constriction of the lower fields cause difficulties in walking around as they are liable to bump into things or trip on steps, stairs or on low furniture. Walking into doorframes is quite common. This can result in either timid behaviour as the child fears accidents or alternatively reckless disregard of danger (as what they can't see won't hurt them!). This is more common in those with high pain thresholds (very common is ASD). Signs that problems are present include clumsiness, eating with hands and difficulties with riding a bike.

In education loss of lower field may result in reading or copying from the board problems. Parents should be aware that the child with a head down posture may be responding to a loss of lower field. Some sports can be a problem, depending on visual demands.

Binocular vision problems are very common in ASD. Almost a half of those on the spectrum will experience some problems but it is important to remember that standard assessment techniques or interventions may not be optimum (or even appropriate) in those with ASD. A high proportion of the binocular vision problems will cease immediately if visual processing interventions are undertaken. The question is – which should be done first – standard binocular interventions or visual processing management. The usual order is standard first, but is this best practice? My own view is that it is sometimes much better to address the processing problems when they appear to be causative but to be aware of the possibility they may be consequential.

This view is somewhat controversial but it may be that as most optical professionals use only the standard techniques, they are unlikely to have seen the differences and will assume that the methods they have been taught are optimum.

Outcomes are usually better if the binocular vision anomaly is treated by processing interventions if it is caused by processing difficulties. These difficulties are usually obvious if looked for. And unlike most traditional methods processing interventions are usually immediately successful. For example some types of squints cannot be addressed using traditional methods – yet resolve immediately using processing methods. Some double vision will only resolve using processing techniques and when visual timing problems are present, the only method of resolving them is to use visual processing interventions.

So, if a binocular vision problem is present what should you do?– it is an extremely difficult choice – my own would be to go somewhere that uses both traditional and processing techniques – at least that way you cover all options.

Assessment techniques

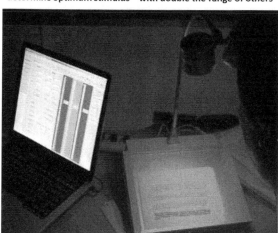

The Orthoscopics Read Eye is the most advanced instrument to determine optimum stimulus – with double the range of others

Stimulus control

We use an additive colour instrument to determine optimum lighting and from that we can utilise some complex maths to determine the best tints and filters. It is based on the principal of univariance and is the most advanced instrument currently available. Tolerances are to within 1 MCAdams ellipse, specifications are to 0.001 XY coordinates CIE 1931 and lenses are to a tolerance of

2.5% LTF. The gamut used for assessment is XY 1931 CIE 0.136/0.056, 0.138.0697, 0.612/0.360

We use the Orthoscopics Read Eye to assess the absolute best colour, with each eye individually and from this can specify the tint for virtually any ambient light. All optical professionals should be able to determine the best filter for a given task. It is an essential part of their professional practice.

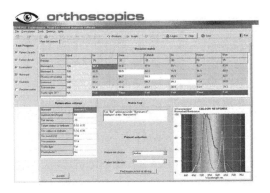

We use a variety of tests depending on presentation and try to show the difference between optimum, normal environment and worst possible (to provoke effects). The improvement possible should be obvious to the child, the parent and to the clinician. It is possible to assess optimum colour for a non- verbal child.

Trial and error techniques can work but there are a number of technical problems with these methods and they are unlikely to give absolute measures. This makes it difficult to replicate lenses unless you use the "sole supplier", which can make them a very expensive solution (although new types of lenses which should be available soon may make this more viable).

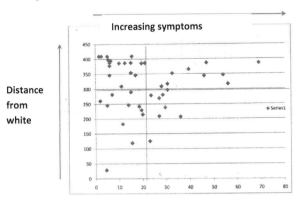

Position in colour space determines potential effects

Treatments will include

Lighting modification – expert knowledge is needed in this area

Spectacles with tints or filters – we use mainly band filters (lenses with sharp colour cut-offs), although broad spectrum (lenses which are designed not to change colour perception much) filters will be effective in some cases. It is essential that the person supplying the filter checks the refractive and optometric effects of the filter as these can modify and inter-relate. It is not a good idea to get your refractive prescription and make the tints in a different practice as there will be inevitable problems which cannot be foreseen. Notch filters (very sharp cut off tints) can be used as a boost.

Tinted lenses are a minefield for the non- expert. Whilst they appear simple they are in fact extremely complex. Some extremely dubious claims are made about tints, and it is fair to say that it is virtually impossible for the average member of the public to be able to work out which are best. In fact with the correct level of knowledge it is possible to work out a variety of tints that can fulfil the task in a specific lighting condition providing there is an absolute prescription of colour space coordinates. Any reputable person will be happy to supply these although you may still find that it is easier to have them supplied where you are tested. But to say that one type of tint manufacture is the best is wrong and if a person says this is true be very careful.

DO NOT TRY AND MATCH A TINT BY EYE – it is virtually impossible for a layman to get right and the effects may be massively different. The tint may also be very different in varying light conditions. Overlays are rarely advised.

Contact lenses

Contact lenses can be used in some cases although it is more difficult to control tints as accurately as in spectacles. Fitting requires clinical knowledge and the tint itself may cause some clinical problems. This is complex and requires an experts input.

The future

Sensory processing problems are very common in ASD. They can cause very unpleasant effects. These should be addressed. Children have a right to see adequately – when it is possible. It is not acceptable for them to be effectively face blind, unable to trust their senses due to their vision or suffering unnecessarily.

If your optical professional cannot or will not address visual processing problems they should refer you to someone that can.

You must question them before attending – the difference between optimum and minimal assessments can change your child's life. You owe it to your child to get optimum assessments and interventions

Training for optical professionals has to change dramatically – they should be able to control visual stimulus and use its effects in ASD – that is their job. But your child needs help now – please make sure they get it!

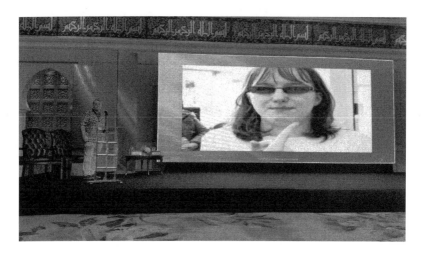

Ian speaking at World Autism Conference 2014

The author

Ian Jordan is a specialist optician in practice in Ayr Scotland. He is an internationally recognised lecturer in the field of tints and filters and their effects (in special needs and other applications) and has written a number of books, designed tints and filters for well- known manufacturers, was the first person to fit contact lenses for dyslexia, has won a number of awards for R&D, made DVD in association with UK university.

He regrets he cannot comment on anyone that he has not seen.

www.jordanseyes.com